DIABETIC TYPE 2 GROCERY AND FOOD LIST

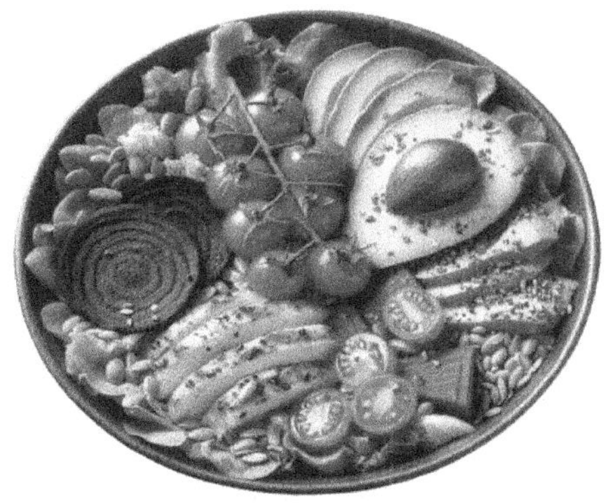

Your Ultimate pocket guide on Low Glycemic Index Nutrition with 30 Delectable and Nutrient-Packed Recipes for Empowering Diabetes Reversal

Tina Feldman

Table of Contents

INTRODUCTION

Type 2 Diabetes is a chronic metabolic condition characterized by the body's inability to effectively use insulin or to produce enough insulin to maintain normal blood sugar levels. Unlike Type 1 Diabetes, which is often diagnosed in childhood and involves the immune system attacking insulin-producing cells, Type 2 Diabetes typically develops in adulthood and is strongly linked to lifestyle factors such as diet, physical activity, and obesity. This prevalent condition affects how the body processes glucose, leading to elevated blood sugar levels.

Managing Type 2 Diabetes involves lifestyle modifications, including a balanced diet, regular exercise, and sometimes medication, to ensure optimal blood sugar control and prevent complications. It is essential for individuals with Type 2 Diabetes to work closely with healthcare professionals to develop a personalized care plan tailored to their specific needs.

Understanding the role of diet in managing Type 2 Diabetes

Understanding the role of diet is paramount in managing Type 2 Diabetes. Diet plays a crucial role in controlling blood sugar levels, managing weight, and reducing the risk of complications associated with diabetes. Here are key aspects to consider when it comes to the diet and managing Type 2 Diabetes:

1. Carbohydrate Management:
   1. Focus on Complex Carbs: Choose whole grains, legumes, and vegetables over refined carbohydrates. These complex carbs have a lower glycemic index, leading to a slower rise in blood sugar levels.
   2. Portion Control: Be mindful of portion sizes to avoid spikes in blood sugar. Balancing carbohydrates throughout the day can help maintain stable glucose levels.

2. Balanced Diet:
   1. Include Protein: Incorporate lean protein sources such as poultry, fish, tofu, and legumes into meals. Protein helps regulate blood sugar and keeps you feeling full.
   2. Healthy Fats: Opt for sources of healthy fats, including avocados, nuts, seeds, and olive oil. These fats can help improve insulin sensitivity.

3. Fiber-Rich Foods:
   1. Emphasize Fiber: Foods high in fiber, such as fruits, vegetables, and whole grains, can help control blood sugar levels and improve digestion. Aim for a variety of colors and types of plant-based foods.

4. Sugar Management:
- Limit Added Sugars: Minimize the intake of foods and drinks with added sugars. Opt for natural sweeteners or limit sweet treats to occasional indulgences.
- Read Labels: Be vigilant about reading food labels to identify hidden sugars and make informed choices.

5. Meal Timing:
- Regular Meals: Aim for regular, balanced meals throughout the day. Spacing meals evenly can help regulate blood sugar levels and prevent overeating.

6. Weight Management:
- Healthy Weight: Achieving and maintaining a healthy weight is essential for managing Type 2 Diabetes. Weight loss, even a modest amount, can improve insulin sensitivity and blood sugar control.

7. Hydration:
- Water Intake: Stay well-hydrated by consuming water throughout the day. Sugary beverages can contribute to blood sugar spikes and should be limited.

8. Consultation with Healthcare Professionals:
- Individualized Approach: Consult with a healthcare team, including a registered dietitian or nutritionist. They can provide

personalized advice based on individual health, lifestyle, and dietary preferences.
- Regular Monitoring: Regularly monitor blood sugar levels and adjust the diet as needed. This can help identify patterns and make informed choices to manage diabetes effectively.

9. Lifestyle Factors:
- Physical Activity: Combine a healthy diet with regular physical activity. Exercise helps improve insulin sensitivity and contributes to overall well-being.
- Stress Management: Manage stress through relaxation techniques, as stress can impact blood sugar levels.

Importance of prioritizing nutrient-rich choices

Prioritizing nutrient-rich choices is of utmost importance for individuals managing Type 2 Diabetes. Nutrient-dense foods provide essential vitamins, minerals, fiber, and other beneficial compounds that support overall health and specifically aid in blood sugar management. Here's a closer look at the importance of prioritizing nutrient-rich choices:

1. Blood Sugar Regulation:
Slow Absorption: Nutrient-rich foods, especially those high in fiber and complex carbohydrates, are absorbed more slowly. This gradual absorption helps

prevent rapid spikes in blood sugar levels, promoting better glycemic control.

2. Weight Management:
Satiety: Nutrient-dense foods are often rich in fiber and protein, promoting a feeling of fullness. This helps in controlling portion sizes and reducing overall calorie intake, contributing to weight management—a crucial aspect for those with Type 2 Diabetes.

3. Heart Health:
Heart-Healthy Nutrients: Nutrient-rich choices, such as fruits, vegetables, whole grains, and fatty fish, contain heart-healthy nutrients like omega-3 fatty acids, potassium, and antioxidants. Managing cardiovascular health is essential for individuals with diabetes, as they are at an increased risk of heart-related complications.

4. Micronutrient Support:
Vitamin and Mineral Intake: Nutrient-dense foods provide essential vitamins and minerals necessary for various bodily functions. These micronutrients play a vital role in supporting immune function, bone health, and overall well-being.

5. Gut Health:
Fiber Content: Many nutrient-rich foods are excellent sources of dietary fiber. Fiber is crucial for maintaining a healthy gut microbiota, which has been linked to improved metabolic health and

reduced inflammation—important considerations for those with Type 2 Diabetes.

6. Reduced Inflammation:
Antioxidant Properties: Nutrient-dense foods, particularly colorful fruits and vegetables, often contain antioxidants that help reduce inflammation. Chronic inflammation is associated with insulin resistance, a key factor in Type 2 Diabetes.

7. Stabilizing Energy Levels:
Balanced Macronutrients: Nutrient-rich choices provide a balance of carbohydrates, proteins, and fats, contributing to stable energy levels throughout the day. This can help prevent energy crashes and overeating.

8. Blood Pressure Management:
Potassium-Rich Foods: Nutrient-dense options, such as bananas, spinach, and sweet potatoes, are high in potassium, which is beneficial for maintaining healthy blood pressure levels—an important consideration for individuals with diabetes.

9. Individualized Nutrition:
Personalized Approach: Nutrient-rich choices allow for a more individualized approach to nutrition, considering specific health needs, preferences, and cultural factors. This flexibility makes it easier for individuals to adhere to a diabetes-friendly diet.

10. Long-Term Health and Prevention:
Disease Prevention: Prioritizing nutrient-rich choices can contribute to the prevention of complications associated with Type 2 Diabetes, such as heart disease, kidney problems, and nerve damage.

BUILDING YOUR GROCERY LIST: ESSENTIAL STAPLE GROUPS

Non-starchy vegetables

Broccoli:
GI: Low
Calories: Approximately 55 per cup (chopped)
Cholesterol: 0 mg
Sugar: 2.4g

Spinach:
GI: Low
Calories: Approximately 7 per cup (raw)
Cholesterol: 0 mg
Sugar: 0.1g

Cauliflower:
GI: Low
Calories: Approximately 27 per cup (chopped)
Cholesterol: 0 mg
Sugar: 2.0g

Zucchini:
GI: Low
Calories: Approximately 20 per cup (sliced)

Cholesterol: 0 mg
Sugar: 2.0g

Bell Peppers (Assorted Colors):
GI: Low
Calories: Approximately 24 per cup (sliced)
Cholesterol: 0 mg
Sugar: 4.2g

Asparagus:
GI: Low
Calories: Approximately 27 per cup (chopped)
Cholesterol: 0 mg
Sugar: 1.9g

Cabbage:
GI: Low
Calories: Approximately 22 per cup (shredded)
Cholesterol: 0 mg
Sugar: 2.3g

Mushrooms:
GI: Low
Calories: Approximately 15 per cup (sliced)
Cholesterol: 0 mg
Sugar: 1.0g

Cucumber:
GI: Low
Calories: Approximately 16 per cup (sliced)
Cholesterol: 0 mg
Sugar: 1.9g

Brussels Sprouts:
GI: Low
Calories: Approximately 38 per cup (cooked)
Cholesterol: 0 mg
Sugar: 1.9g

Green Beans:
GI: Low
Calories: Approximately 31 per cup (cooked)
Cholesterol: 0 mg
Sugar: 3.6g

Kale:
GI: Low
Calories: Approximately 34 per cup (chopped)
Cholesterol: 0 mg
Sugar: 0.6g

Eggplant:
GI: Low
Calories: Approximately 20 per cup (cubed)
Cholesterol: 0 mg
Sugar: 2.5g

Onions:
GI: Low
Calories: Approximately 64 per cup (chopped)
Cholesterol: 0 mg
Sugar: 6.0g

Tomatoes:
GI: Low to moderate
Calories: Approximately 32 per cup (chopped)

Cholesterol: 0 mg
Sugar: 4.0g

Protein sources

Chicken Breast (Skinless, Boneless):
Calories: Approximately 165 per 3.5 oz (cooked)
Cholesterol: 73 mg
Sugar: 0g

Salmon (Wild-caught):
Calories: Approximately 206 per 3.5 oz (cooked)
Cholesterol: 63 mg
Sugar: 0g

Turkey (Ground, Lean):
Calories: Approximately 220 per 3.5 oz (cooked)
Cholesterol: 70 mg
Sugar: 0g

Tofu:
Calories: Approximately 94 per 3.5 oz (raw)
Cholesterol: 0 mg
Sugar: 0.3g

Eggs:
Calories: Approximately 68 per large egg (boiled)
Cholesterol: 186 mg
Sugar: 0.6g

Greek Yogurt (Plain, Non-fat):
Calories: Approximately 59 per 100g
Cholesterol: 10 mg

Sugar: 4.0g

Cottage Cheese (Low-fat):
Calories: Approximately 206 per cup
Cholesterol: 14 mg
Sugar: 6.0g

Beans (Black Beans):
Calories: Approximately 114 per 3.5 oz (cooked)
Cholesterol: 0 mg
Sugar: 0.3g

Lentils:
Calories: Approximately 165 per cup (cooked)
Cholesterol: 0 mg
Sugar: 3.3g

Chickpeas:
Calories: Approximately 164 per cup (cooked)
Cholesterol: 0 mg
Sugar: 4.8g

Lean Beef (Sirloin):
Calories: Approximately 250 per 3.5 oz (cooked)
Cholesterol: 95 mg
Sugar: 0g

Pork Tenderloin:
Calories: Approximately 143 per 3.5 oz (cooked)
Cholesterol: 63 mg
Sugar: 0g

Quinoa:
Calories: Approximately 222 per cup (cooked)
Cholesterol: 0 mg
Sugar: 0.9g

Almonds:
Calories: Approximately 206 per 1 oz
Cholesterol: 0 mg
Sugar: 1.0g

Soy Milk (Unsweetened):
Calories: Approximately 33 per cup
Cholesterol: 0 mg
Sugar: 0.2g

Healthy fats

Avocado:
Calories: Approximately 234 per avocado
Cholesterol: 0 mg
Sugar: 0.2g

Olive Oil:
Calories: Approximately 120 per tablespoon
Cholesterol: 0 mg
Sugar: 0g

Salmon (Fatty Fish):
Calories: Approximately 206 per 3.5 oz (cooked)
Cholesterol: 63 mg
Sugar: 0g

Nuts (Almonds):
Calories: Approximately 206 per 1 oz

Cholesterol: 0 mg
Sugar: 1.0g

Chia Seeds:
Calories: Approximately 138 per 2 tablespoons
Cholesterol: 0 mg
Sugar: 0g

Flaxseeds:
Calories: Approximately 150 per 2 tablespoons
Cholesterol: 0 mg
Sugar: 0.2g

Walnuts:
Calories: Approximately 185 per 1 oz
Cholesterol: 0 mg
Sugar: 0.7g

Coconut Oil:
Calories: Approximately 120 per tablespoon
Cholesterol: 0 mg
Sugar: 0g

Dark Chocolate (70-85% cocoa):
Calories: Approximately 170 per 1 oz
Cholesterol: 0 mg
Sugar: 2.0g

Peanut Butter (Natural, No Added Sugar):
Calories: Approximately 190 per 2 tablespoons
Cholesterol: 0 mg
Sugar: 1.0g

Hummus (Chickpea-based):
Calories: Approximately 70 per 2 tablespoons
Cholesterol: 0 mg
Sugar: 0.2g

Sesame Oil:
Calories: Approximately 120 per tablespoon
Cholesterol: 0 mg
Sugar: 0g

Sunflower Seeds:
Calories: Approximately 180 per 1 oz
Cholesterol: 0 mg
Sugar: 0.5g

Fatty Fish (Mackerel):
Calories: Approximately 305 per 3.5 oz (cooked)
Cholesterol: 90 mg
Sugar: 0g

Edamame (Soybeans):
Calories: Approximately 120 per cup (cooked)
Cholesterol: 0 mg
Sugar: 3.5g

Quinoa:
Calories: Approximately 222 per cup (cooked)
Cholesterol: 0 mg
Sugar: 0.9g

Brown Rice:
Calories: Approximately 215 per cup (cooked)
Cholesterol: 0 mg
Sugar: 0.7g

Oats (Old-fashioned):
Calories: Approximately 154 per 1/2 cup (uncooked)
Cholesterol: 0 mg
Sugar: 1.0g

Barley:
Calories: Approximately 193 per cup (cooked)
Cholesterol: 0 mg
Sugar: 0.8g

Bulgur:
Calories: Approximately 151 per cup (cooked)
Cholesterol: 0 mg
Sugar: 0.4g

Whole Wheat Pasta:
Calories: Approximately 174 per cup (cooked)
Cholesterol: 0 mg
Sugar: 1.1g

Millet:
Calories: Approximately 207 per cup (cooked)
Cholesterol: 0 mg
Sugar: 0.4g

Farro:
Calories: Approximately 337 per cup (cooked)
Cholesterol: 0 mg
Sugar: 0.4g

Whole Wheat Bread:
Calories: Approximately 69 per slice (28g)
Cholesterol: 0 mg
Sugar: 1.0g

Buckwheat:
Calories: Approximately 155 per cup (cooked)
Cholesterol: 0 mg
Sugar: 0.6g

Rye:
Calories: Approximately 150 per 1 ounce (uncooked)
Cholesterol: 0 mg
Sugar: 0g

Sorghum:
Calories: Approximately 339 per cup (cooked)
Cholesterol: 0 mg
Sugar: 0g

Wild Rice:
Calories: Approximately 166 per cup (cooked)
Cholesterol: 0 mg
Sugar: 0.7g

Whole Wheat Tortillas:
Calories: Approximately 104 per 1 tortilla (49g)
Cholesterol: 0 mg
Sugar: 0.7g

Amaranth:
Calories: Approximately 251 per cup (cooked)
Cholesterol: 0 mg
Sugar: 1.6g

Low-fat dairy or alternatives

Greek Yogurt (Low-fat, Unsweetened):
Calories: Approximately 59 per 100g
Cholesterol: 10 mg
Sugar: 4.0g

Skim Milk:
Calories: Approximately 86 per cup
Cholesterol: 5 mg
Sugar: 12.3g

Low-fat Cottage Cheese:
Calories: Approximately 206 per cup
Cholesterol: 14 mg
Sugar: 6.0g

Almond Milk (Unsweetened):
Calories: Approximately 13 per cup
Cholesterol: 0 mg
Sugar: 0g

Low-fat Mozzarella Cheese:
Calories: Approximately 71 per ounce
Cholesterol: 15 mg
Sugar: 0.1g

Low-fat Ricotta Cheese:
Calories: Approximately 39 per ounce
Cholesterol: 14 mg
Sugar: 0.4g

Low-fat Swiss Cheese:
Calories: Approximately 50 per slice (1 oz)
Cholesterol: 20 mg
Sugar: 0.1g

Soy Milk (Unsweetened):
Calories: Approximately 33 per cup
Cholesterol: 0 mg
Sugar: 0.2g

Low-fat Plain Kefir:
Calories: Approximately 110 per cup
Cholesterol: 10 mg
Sugar: 12.0g

Low-fat Yogurt (Flavored, No Added Sugar):
Calories: Approximately 150 per cup
Cholesterol: 15 mg

Sugar: 6.0g

Low-fat String Cheese:
Calories: Approximately 50 per piece
Cholesterol: 15 mg
Sugar: 0g

Coconut Milk (Unsweetened):
Calories: Approximately 50 per cup
Cholesterol: 0 mg
Sugar: 0g

Low-fat Buttermilk:
Calories: Approximately 98 per cup
Cholesterol: 12 mg
Sugar: 11.7g

Low-fat Sour Cream:
Calories: Approximately 46 per 2 tablespoons
Cholesterol: 14 mg
Sugar: 1.0g

Low-fat Cream Cheese:
Calories: Approximately 30 per 2 tablespoons
Cholesterol: 10 mg
Sugar: 1.0g

Fruits: Low-glycemic options

Berries (Strawberries):
Calories: Approximately 49 per cup
Cholesterol: 0 mg
Sugar: 7.4g

Cherries:
Calories: Approximately 87 per cup (pitted)
Cholesterol: 0 mg
Sugar: 18.9g

Grapefruit (Pink):
Calories: Approximately 52 per medium fruit
Cholesterol: 0 mg
Sugar: 8.9g

Apples (with skin):
Calories: Approximately 95 per medium apple
Cholesterol: 0 mg
Sugar: 19.0g

Pears (with skin):
Calories: Approximately 101 per medium pear
Cholesterol: 0 mg
Sugar: 17.3g

Peaches:
Calories: Approximately 59 per medium peach
Cholesterol: 0 mg
Sugar: 13.1g

Plums:
Calories: Approximately 30 per medium plum
Cholesterol: 0 mg
Sugar: 6.3g

Apricots:
Calories: Approximately 17 per apricot
Cholesterol: 0 mg
Sugar: 3.9g

Kiwi:
Calories: Approximately 61 per medium kiwi
Cholesterol: 0 mg
Sugar: 9.0g

Oranges:
Calories: Approximately 62 per medium orange
Cholesterol: 0 mg
Sugar: 12.2g

Cantaloupe:
Calories: Approximately 53 per cup (cubed)
Cholesterol: 0 mg
Sugar: 12.3g

Nectarines:
Calories: Approximately 62 per medium nectarine
Cholesterol: 0 mg
Sugar: 11.3g

Raspberries:
Calories: Approximately 65 per cup
Cholesterol: 0 mg

Sugar: 5.4g

Blackberries:
Calories: Approximately 62 per cup
Cholesterol: 0 mg
Sugar: 7.0g

Watermelon:
Calories: Approximately 46 per cup (cubed)
Cholesterol: 0 mg
Sugar: 9.4g

Sweeteners

Stevia:
Calories: Negligible
Cholesterol: 0 mg
Sugar: 0g

Monk Fruit Sweetener:
Calories: Negligible
Cholesterol: 0 mg
Sugar: 0g

Erythritol:
Calories: Approximately 0.24 per gram
Cholesterol: 0 mg
Sugar: 0g

Xylitol:
Calories: Approximately 2.4 per gram
Cholesterol: 0 mg
Sugar: 0g

Agave Nectar (in moderation):
Calories: Approximately 60 per tablespoon
Cholesterol: 0 mg
Sugar: 16.0g

Coconut Sugar:
Calories: Approximately 15 per teaspoon
Cholesterol: 0 mg
Sugar: 4.0g

Allulose:
Calories: Approximately 0.2 per gram
Cholesterol: 0 mg
Sugar: 0g

Sucralose (Splenda):
Calories: Negligible
Cholesterol: 0 mg
Sugar: 0g

Aspartame:
Calories: Negligible
Cholesterol: 0 mg
Sugar: 0g

Saccharin (Sweet'N Low):
Calories: Negligible
Cholesterol: 0 mg
Sugar: 0g

Neotame:
Calories: Negligible
Cholesterol: 0 mg

Sugar: 0g

Tagatose:
Calories: Approximately 1.5 per gram
Cholesterol: 0 mg
Sugar: 2.0g

Maltitol:
Calories: Approximately 2.1 per gram
Cholesterol: 0 mg
Sugar: 0g

Sorbitol:
Calories: Approximately 2.6 per gram
Cholesterol: 0 mg
Sugar: 0g

Brown Rice Syrup:
Calories: Approximately 55 per tablespoon
Cholesterol: 0 mg
Sugar: 7.3g

Raw Almonds:
Calories: Approximately 160 per ounce
Cholesterol: 0 mg
Sugar: 1.0g

Baby Carrots with Hummus:
Calories: Approximately 50 (1 cup of baby carrots +
2 tablespoons of hummus)
Cholesterol: 0 mg
Sugar: 2.0g

Greek Yogurt with Berries:
Calories: Approximately 150 per serving (6 oz)
Cholesterol: 10 mg
Sugar: 8.0g

String Cheese:
Calories: Approximately 80 per piece
Cholesterol: 15 mg
Sugar: 0g

Hard-Boiled Eggs:
Calories: Approximately 68 per large egg
Cholesterol: 186 mg
Sugar: 0.6g

Celery Sticks with Peanut Butter (Natural, No Added
Sugar):
Calories: Approximately 100 (2 medium celery
sticks + 2 tablespoons peanut butter)
Cholesterol: 0 mg
Sugar: 2.0g

Cherry Tomatoes with Mozzarella Cheese:
Calories: Approximately 100 (1 cup cherry tomatoes + 1 ounce mozzarella)
Cholesterol: 20 mg
Sugar: 3.0g

Whole Grain Crackers with Sliced Turkey:
Calories: Approximately 150 (6 whole grain crackers + 2 oz turkey)
Cholesterol: 40 mg
Sugar: 0g

Cottage Cheese with Pineapple Chunks (in juice, no added sugar):
Calories: Approximately 150 per cup
Cholesterol: 14 mg
Sugar: 8.0g

Avocado Slices with Cherry Tomatoes:
Calories: Approximately 120 (1/2 avocado + 1 cup cherry tomatoes)
Cholesterol: 0 mg
Sugar: 2.0g

Seeds (Pumpkin or Sunflower):
Calories: Approximately 180 per ounce
Cholesterol: 0 mg
Sugar: 0g

Beef Jerky (Low-sodium, No Added Sugar):
Calories: Approximately 80 per 1 ounce
Cholesterol: 20 mg
Sugar: 1.0g

Apple Slices with Almond Butter (Natural, No Added Sugar):
Calories: Approximately 200 (1 medium apple + 2 tablespoons almond butter)
Cholesterol: 0 mg
Sugar: 12.0g

Air-Popped Popcorn:
Calories: Approximately 31 per cup
Cholesterol: 0 mg
Sugar: 0g

Vegetable Sticks (Cucumber, Bell Pepper) with Guacamole:
Calories: Approximately 150 (1 cup vegetable sticks + 2 tablespoons guacamole)
Cholesterol: 0 mg
Sugar: 3.0g

Legumes

Chickpeas (Garbanzo Beans):
Calories: Approximately 164 per cup (cooked)
Cholesterol: 0 mg
Sugar: 2.6g

Black Beans:
Calories: Approximately 227 per cup (cooked)
Cholesterol: 0 mg
Sugar: 0.6g

Lentils:
Calories: Approximately 230 per cup (cooked)
Cholesterol: 0 mg

Sugar: 0.8g

Kidney Beans:
Calories: Approximately 215 per cup (cooked)
Cholesterol: 0 mg
Sugar: 0.3g

Pinto Beans:
Calories: Approximately 245 per cup (cooked)
Cholesterol: 0 mg
Sugar: 0.6g

Cannellini Beans:
Calories: Approximately 224 per cup (cooked)
Cholesterol: 0 mg
Sugar: 0.5g

Split Peas:
Calories: Approximately 231 per cup (cooked)
Cholesterol: 0 mg
Sugar: 0.8g

Black-eyed Peas:
Calories: Approximately 198 per cup (cooked)
Cholesterol: 0 mg
Sugar: 0.6g

Garlic Hummus:
Calories: Approximately 27 per tablespoon
Cholesterol: 0 mg
Sugar: 0.2g

Edamame:
Calories: Approximately 189 per cup (cooked)
Cholesterol: 0 mg
Sugar: 2.2g

Chana Dal (Split Chickpeas):
Calories: Approximately 160 per cup (cooked)
Cholesterol: 0 mg
Sugar: 1.6g

Green Peas:
Calories: Approximately 62 per 1/2 cup (cooked)
Cholesterol: 0 mg
Sugar: 4.5g

Adzuki Beans:
Calories: Approximately 294 per cup (cooked)
Cholesterol: 0 mg
Sugar: 0.2g

Mung Beans:
Calories: Approximately 212 per cup (cooked)
Cholesterol: 0 mg
Sugar: 1.4g

Red Lentils:
Calories: Approximately 230 per cup (cooked)
Cholesterol: 0 mg
Sugar: 1.0g

Low glycemic vegetables

Broccoli:
Calories: Approximately 55 per cup (chopped)
GI: Low
GL: Low
Sugar: 2.4g

Spinach:
Calories: Approximately 7 per cup (raw)
GI: Low
GL: Low
Sugar: 0.1g

Cauliflower:
Calories: Approximately 27 per cup (chopped)
GI: Low
GL: Low
Sugar: 2.0g

Zucchini:
Calories: Approximately 20 per cup (sliced)
GI: Low
GL: Low
Sugar: 2.0g

Bell Peppers (Assorted Colors):
Calories: Approximately 24 per cup (sliced)

GI: Low
GL: Low
Sugar: 4.2g

Asparagus:
Calories: Approximately 27 per cup (chopped)
GI: Low
GL: Low
Sugar: 1.9g

Cabbage:
Calories: Approximately 22 per cup (shredded)
GI: Low
GL: Low
Sugar: 2.3g

Mushrooms:
Calories: Approximately 15 per cup (sliced)
GI: Low
GL: Low
Sugar: 1.0g

Cucumber:
Calories: Approximately 16 per cup (sliced)
GI: Low
GL: Low
Sugar: 1.9g

Brussels Sprouts:
Calories: Approximately 38 per cup (cooked)

GI: Low
GL: Low
Sugar: 1.9g

Green Beans:
Calories: Approximately 31 per cup (cooked)
GI: Low
GL: Low
Sugar: 3.6g

Kale:
Calories: Approximately 34 per cup (chopped)
GI: Low
GL: Low
Sugar: 0.6g

Eggplant:
Calories: Approximately 20 per cup (cubed)
GI: Low
GL: Low
Sugar: 2.5g

Onions:
Calories: Approximately 64 per cup (chopped)
GI: Low
GL: Low
Sugar: 6.0g

Tomatoes:
Calories: Approximately 32 per cup (chopped)

GI: Low to moderate
GL: Low
Sugar: 4.0g

Low glycemic whole grains

Quinoa:
Calories: Approximately 222 per cup (cooked)
GI: Low to moderate
GL: Low
Sugar: 0.9g

Brown Rice:
Calories: Approximately 215 per cup (cooked)
GI: Low to moderate
GL: Low
Sugar: 0.7g

Steel-Cut Oats:
Calories: Approximately 150 per 1/4 cup (dry)
GI: Low to moderate
GL: Low
Sugar: 0.5g

Barley:
Calories: Approximately 193 per cup (cooked)
GI: Low to moderate
GL: Low
Sugar: 0.8g

Bulgur:
Calories: Approximately 151 per cup (cooked)

GI: Low to moderate
GL: Low
Sugar: 0.4g

Whole Wheat Pasta:
Calories: Approximately 174 per cup (cooked)
GI: Low to moderate
GL: Low
Sugar: 1.1g

Millet:
Calories: Approximately 207 per cup (cooked)
GI: Low to moderate
GL: Low
Sugar: 0.4g

Farro:
Calories: Approximately 337 per cup (cooked)
GI: Low to moderate
GL: Low
Sugar: 0.4g

Quinoa Pasta:
Calories: Varies by brand, refer to product label
GI: Low to moderate
GL: Low
Sugar: Varies by brand

Whole Wheat Bread:
Calories: Approximately 69 per slice (28g)

GI: Low to moderate
GL: Low
Sugar: 1.0g

Buckwheat:
Calories: Approximately 155 per cup (cooked)
GI: Low to moderate
GL: Low
Sugar: 0.6g

Rye Bread:
Calories: Varies by brand, refer to product label
GI: Low to moderate
GL: Low
Sugar: Varies by brand

Sorghum:
Calories: Approximately 339 per cup (cooked)
GI: Low to moderate
GL: Low
Sugar: 0g

Wild Rice:
Calories: Approximately 166 per cup (cooked)
GI: Low to moderate
GL: Low
Sugar: 0.7g

Amaranth:
Calories: Approximately 251 per cup (cooked)

GI: Low to moderate
GL: Low
Sugar: 1.6g

Low glycemic fruits

Berries (Strawberries):
Calories: Approximately 49 per cup
GI: Low
GL: Low
Sugar: 7.4g

Cherries:
Calories: Approximately 87 per cup (pitted)
GI: Low to moderate
GL: Low
Sugar: 18.9g

Grapefruit (Pink):
Calories: Approximately 52 per medium fruit
GI: Low to moderate
GL: Low
Sugar: 8.9g

Apples (with skin):
Calories: Approximately 95 per medium apple
GI: Low to moderate
GL: Low
Sugar: 19.0g

Pears (with skin):
Calories: Approximately 101 per medium pear

GI: Low to moderate
GL: Low
Sugar: 17.3g

Peaches:
Calories: Approximately 59 per medium peach
GI: Low to moderate
GL: Low
Sugar: 13.1g

Plums:
Calories: Approximately 30 per medium plum
GI: Low to moderate
GL: Low
Sugar: 6.3g

Apricots:
Calories: Approximately 17 per apricot
GI: Low to moderate
GL: Low
Sugar: 3.9g

Kiwi:
Calories: Approximately 61 per medium kiwi
GI: Low to moderate
GL: Low
Sugar: 9.0g

Oranges:
Calories: Approximately 62 per medium orange

GI: Low to moderate
GL: Low
Sugar: 12.2g

Cantaloupe:
Calories: Approximately 53 per cup (cubed)
GI: Low to moderate
GL: Low
Sugar: 12.3g

Nectarines:
Calories: Approximately 62 per medium nectarine
GI: Low to moderate
GL: Low
Sugar: 11.3g

Raspberries:
Calories: Approximately 65 per cup
GI: Low
GL: Low
Sugar: 5.4g

Blackberries:
Calories: Approximately 62 per cup
GI: Low
GL: Low
Sugar: 7.0g

Watermelon:
Calories: Approximately 46 per cup (cubed)

GI: Low to moderate
GL: Low
Sugar: 9.4g

Low glycemic soup and broth

Chicken Broth (Low-sodium):
Calories: Varies by brand, refer to product label
GI: Low
GL: Low
Sugar: Varies by brand

Vegetable Broth (Low-sodium):
Calories: Varies by brand, refer to product label
GI: Low
GL: Low
Sugar: Varies by brand

Beef Broth (Low-sodium):
Calories: Varies by brand, refer to product label
GI: Low
GL: Low
Sugar: Varies by brand

Tomato Soup (No Added Sugar):
Calories: Varies by brand, refer to product label
GI: Low to moderate
GL: Low to moderate
Sugar: Varies by brand

Mushroom Soup (Low-sodium):
Calories: Varies by brand, refer to product label

GI: Low to moderate
GL: Low to moderate
Sugar: Varies by brand

Lentil Soup (Low-sodium):
Calories: Varies by brand, refer to product label
GI: Low to moderate
GL: Low to moderate
Sugar: Varies by brand

Minestrone Soup (Low-sodium):
Calories: Varies by brand, refer to product label
GI: Low to moderate
GL: Low to moderate
Sugar: Varies by brand

Chicken and Vegetable Soup (Low-sodium):
Calories: Varies by brand, refer to product label
GI: Low to moderate
GL: Low to moderate
Sugar: Varies by brand

Split Pea Soup (Low-sodium):
Calories: Varies by brand, refer to product label
GI: Low to moderate
GL: Low to moderate
Sugar: Varies by brand

Black Bean Soup (Low-sodium):
Calories: Varies by brand, refer to product label

GI: Low to moderate
GL: Low to moderate
Sugar: Varies by brand

Clam Chowder (Low-sodium):
Calories: Varies by brand, refer to product label
GI: Low to moderate
GL: Low to moderate
Sugar: Varies by brand

Butternut Squash Soup (No Added Sugar):
Calories: Varies by brand, refer to product label
GI: Low to moderate
GL: Low to moderate
Sugar: Varies by brand

Gazpacho (No Added Sugar):
Calories: Varies by brand, refer to product label
GI: Low to moderate
GL: Low to moderate
Sugar: Varies by brand

Cabbage Soup (Low-sodium):
Calories: Varies by recipe, refer to product label
GI: Low to moderate
GL: Low to moderate
Sugar: Varies by recipe

Turkey Chili (Low-sodium):
Calories: Varies by brand, refer to product label

GI: Low to moderate
GL: Low to moderate
Sugar: Varies by brand

Low glycemic legumes and pulse

Chickpeas (Garbanzo Beans):
Calories: Approximately 164 per cup (cooked)
GI: Low
GL: Low
Sugar: 2.6g

Black Beans:
Calories: Approximately 227 per cup (cooked)
GI: Low to moderate
GL: Low
Sugar: 0.6g

Lentils:
Calories: Approximately 230 per cup (cooked)
GI: Low to moderate
GL: Low
Sugar: 0.8g

Kidney Beans:
Calories: Approximately 215 per cup (cooked)
GI: Low to moderate
GL: Low
Sugar: 0.3g

Pinto Beans:
Calories: Approximately 245 per cup (cooked)

GI: Low to moderate
GL: Low
Sugar: 0.6g

Cannellini Beans:
Calories: Approximately 224 per cup (cooked)
GI: Low to moderate
GL: Low
Sugar: 0.5g

Split Peas:
Calories: Approximately 231 per cup (cooked)
GI: Low to moderate
GL: Low
Sugar: 0.8g

Black-eyed Peas:
Calories: Approximately 198 per cup (cooked)
GI: Low to moderate
GL: Low
Sugar: 0.6g

Garlic Hummus:
Calories: Approximately 27 per tablespoon
GI: Low
GL: Low
Sugar: 0.2g

Edamame:
Calories: Approximately 189 per cup (cooked)

GI: Low to moderate
GL: Low
Sugar: 2.2g

Chana Dal (Split Chickpeas):
Calories: Approximately 160 per cup (cooked)
GI: Low
GL: Low
Sugar: 1.6g

Green Peas:
Calories: Approximately 62 per 1/2 cup (cooked)
GI: Low to moderate
GL: Low
Sugar: 4.5g

Adzuki Beans:
Calories: Approximately 294 per cup (cooked)
GI: Low to moderate
GL: Low
Sugar: 0.2g

Mung Beans:
Calories: Approximately 212 per cup (cooked)
GI: Low to moderate
GL: Low
Sugar: 1.4g

Red Lentils:
Calories: Approximately 230 per cup (cooked)

GI: Low to moderate
GL: Low
Sugar: 1.0g

Low glycemic seafood

Salmon:
Calories: Approximately 206 per 3-ounce fillet
Protein: 22g
Fat: 13g
Carbohydrates: 0g
Sugar: 0g

Tuna (canned in water):
Calories: Approximately 179 per cup
Protein: 42g
Fat: 1g
Carbohydrates: 0g
Sugar: 0g

Shrimp:
Calories: Approximately 84 per 3-ounce serving
(cooked)
Protein: 18g
Fat: 1g
Carbohydrates: 0g
Sugar: 0g

Mackerel:
Calories: Approximately 360 per fillet (3.5 ounces)
Protein: 32g
Fat: 25g
Carbohydrates: 0g
Sugar: 0g

Sardines (canned in water):
Calories: Approximately 191 per cup
Protein: 25g
Fat: 10g
Carbohydrates: 0g
Sugar: 0g

Halibut:
Calories: Approximately 158 per 3-ounce fillet
Protein: 23g
Fat: 7g
Carbohydrates: 0g
Sugar: 0g

Cod:
Calories: Approximately 189 per 3-ounce fillet
Protein: 19g
Fat: 1g
Carbohydrates: 0g
Sugar: 0g

Trout:
Calories: Approximately 148 per 3-ounce fillet
Protein: 20g
Fat: 7g
Carbohydrates: 0g
Sugar: 0g

Scallops:

Calories: Approximately 95 per 3-ounce serving (cooked)
Protein: 19g
Fat: 1g
Carbohydrates: 2g
Sugar: 0g

Crab:
Calories: Approximately 98 per 3-ounce serving (cooked)
Protein: 20g
Fat: 1g
Carbohydrates: 0g
Sugar: 0g

Lobster:
Calories: Approximately 129 per 3-ounce serving (cooked)
Protein: 27g
Fat: 1g
Carbohydrates: 1g
Sugar: 0g

Clams:
Calories: Approximately 126 per 3-ounce serving (cooked)
Protein: 22g
Fat: 2g
Carbohydrates: 5g
Sugar: 0g

Oysters:

Calories: Approximately 68 per 3-ounce serving (cooked)
Protein: 9g
Fat: 2g
Carbohydrates: 4g
Sugar: 0g

Tilapia:
Calories: Approximately 111 per 3-ounce fillet
Protein: 23g
Fat: 2g
Carbohydrates: 0g
Sugar: 0g

Canned Anchovies:
Calories: Approximately 131 per 3-ounce can
Protein: 20g
Fat: 5g
Carbohydrates: 0g
Sugar: 0g

Low glycemic protein sources

Chicken Breast:
Calories: Approximately 165 per 3-ounce serving
(cooked)
Protein: 31g
Fat: 3.6g
Carbohydrates: 0g
Sugar: 0g

Turkey (Ground, Lean):
Calories: Approximately 93 per 3-ounce serving
(cooked)
Protein: 19g
Fat: 1.3g
Carbohydrates: 0g
Sugar: 0g

Eggs:
Calories: Approximately 70 per large egg
Protein: 6g
Fat: 5g
Carbohydrates: 1g
Sugar: 1g

Salmon:
Calories: Approximately 206 per 3-ounce fillet
(cooked)
Protein: 22g
Fat: 13g
Carbohydrates: 0g
Sugar: 0g

Tofu:
Calories: Approximately 94 per 3-ounce serving (raw)
Protein: 10g
Fat: 6g
Carbohydrates: 2g
Sugar: 0g

Greek Yogurt (Plain, Non-fat):
Calories: Approximately 100 per 6-ounce serving
Protein: 15g
Fat: 0g
Carbohydrates: 6g
Sugar: 4g

Cottage Cheese (Low-fat):
Calories: Approximately 220 per cup
Protein: 28g
Fat: 10g
Carbohydrates: 8g
Sugar: 6g

Lentils:
Calories: Approximately 230 per cup (cooked)
Protein: 18g
Fat: 0.8g
Carbohydrates: 40g
Sugar: 3.6g

Chickpeas (Garbanzo Beans):
Calories: Approximately 164 per cup (cooked)
Protein: 14.5g
Fat: 2.6g

Carbohydrates: 27g
Sugar: 4.8g

Pumpkin Seeds (Pepitas):
Calories: Approximately 180 per ounce
Protein: 9g
Fat: 15g
Carbohydrates: 4g
Sugar: 0g

Canned Tuna (in water):
Calories: Approximately 179 per cup
Protein: 42g
Fat: 1g
Carbohydrates: 0g
Sugar: 0g

Quinoa:
Calories: Approximately 222 per cup (cooked)
Protein: 8g
Fat: 4g
Carbohydrates: 39g
Sugar: 1.6g

Edamame:
Calories: Approximately 189 per cup (cooked)
Protein: 17g
Fat: 8g
Carbohydrates: 16g
Sugar: 3.3g

Lean Beef (Top Sirloin):
Calories: Approximately 205 per 3-ounce serving
(cooked)
Protein: 26g
Fat: 11g
Carbohydrates: 0g
Sugar: 0g

Canned Salmon (Pink, Wild-caught):
Calories: Approximately 180 per 3-ounce serving
(canned)
Protein: 25g
Fat: 9g
Carbohydrates: 0g
Sugar: 0g

Low glycemic Dairy and Dairy Alternatives

Greek Yogurt (Plain, Non-fat):
Calories: Approximately 100 per 6-ounce serving
Protein: 15g
Fat: 0g
Carbohydrates: 6g
Sugar: 4g

Cottage Cheese (Low-fat):
Calories: Approximately 220 per cup
Protein: 28g
Fat: 10g
Carbohydrates: 8g
Sugar: 6g

Skim Milk:
Calories: Approximately 80 per cup
Protein: 8g
Fat: 0g
Carbohydrates: 12g
Sugar: 12g (natural sugars from lactose)

Almond Milk (Unsweetened):
Calories: Approximately 30 per cup
Protein: 1g
Fat: 2.5g
Carbohydrates: 1g
Sugar: 0g

Coconut Milk (Unsweetened):
Calories: Approximately 45 per cup
Protein: 0g
Fat: 4.5g
Carbohydrates: 1g
Sugar: 0g

Soy Milk (Unsweetened):
Calories: Approximately 80 per cup
Protein: 7g
Fat: 4g
Carbohydrates: 4g
Sugar: 1g

Low-fat Cheese (e.g., Mozzarella):
Calories: Varies by type, refer to product label
Protein: Varies
Fat: Varies
Carbohydrates: Varies

Sugar: Varies

Feta Cheese (Reduced Fat):
Calories: Varies by type, refer to product label
Protein: Varies
Fat: Varies
Carbohydrates: Varies
Sugar: Varies

Plain Yogurt (Non-fat):
Calories: Approximately 150 per cup
Protein: 13g
Fat: 0g
Carbohydrates: 17g
Sugar: 13g (natural sugars from lactose)

Swiss Cheese (Reduced Fat):
Calories: Varies by type, refer to product label
Protein: Varies
Fat: Varies
Carbohydrates: Varies
Sugar: Varies

String Cheese (Part-skim):
Calories: Varies by brand, refer to product label
Protein: Varies
Fat: Varies
Carbohydrates: Varies
Sugar: Varies

Probiotic Yogurt Drink (Unsweetened):
Calories: Approximately 60 per 8-ounce serving
Protein: 5g
Fat: 3g
Carbohydrates: 4g
Sugar: 3g

Ricotta Cheese (Part-skim):
Calories: Approximately 337 per cup
Protein: 14g
Fat: 20g
Carbohydrates: 13g
Sugar: 0g

Cashew Milk (Unsweetened):
Calories: Approximately 25 per cup
Protein: 0.5g
Fat: 2g
Carbohydrates: 1g
Sugar: 0g

Oat Milk (Unsweetened):
Calories: Approximately 80 per cup
Protein: 3g
Fat: 1.5g
Carbohydrates: 15g
Sugar: 0g

Low glycemic nuts and seeds

Almonds:
Calories: Approximately 7 calories per almond
Protein: 0.3g
Fat: 0.6g
Carbohydrates: 0.2g
Sugar: 0g

Walnuts:
Calories: Approximately 4 calories per walnut half
Protein: 0.9g
Fat: 1.9g
Carbohydrates: 0.2g
Sugar: 0g

Pistachios:
Calories: Approximately 4 calories per pistachio
Protein: 0.2g
Fat: 0.3g
Carbohydrates: 0.2g
Sugar: 0.1g

Brazil Nuts:
Calories: Approximately 19 calories per nut
Protein: 0.5g
Fat: 1.9g
Carbohydrates: 0.3g
Sugar: 0g

Cashews:
Calories: Approximately 8 calories per cashew
Protein: 0.3g
Fat: 0.6g

Carbohydrates: 0.1g
Sugar: 0g

Flaxseeds:
Calories: Approximately 37 calories per tablespoon (ground)
Protein: 1.3g
Fat: 3g
Carbohydrates: 1.9g
Sugar: 0.1g

Chia Seeds:
Calories: Approximately 69 calories per ounce
Protein: 2.5g
Fat: 4.4g
Carbohydrates: 5.6g
Sugar: 0.2g

Sunflower Seeds:
Calories: Approximately 6 calories per seed
Protein: 0.3g
Fat: 0.5g
Carbohydrates: 0.2g
Sugar: 0g

Pumpkin Seeds (Pepitas):
Calories: Approximately 7 calories per seed
Protein: 0.3g
Fat: 0.6g
Carbohydrates: 0.2g
Sugar: 0g

Hazelnuts:
Calories: Approximately 9 calories per hazelnut
Protein: 0.2g
Fat: 0.9g
Carbohydrates: 0.3g
Sugar: 0g

Macadamia Nuts:
Calories: Approximately 7 calories per macadamia
nut
Protein: 0.1g
Fat: 0.7g
Carbohydrates: 0.1g
Sugar: 0g

Sesame Seeds:
Calories: Approximately 5 calories per teaspoon
Protein: 0.2g
Fat: 0.4g
Carbohydrates: 0.1g
Sugar: 0g

Almond Butter (No Added Sugar):
Calories: Varies by brand, refer to product label
Protein: Varies
Fat: Varies
Carbohydrates: Varies
Sugar: Varies

Peanut Butter (No Added Sugar):
Calories: Varies by brand, refer to product label
Protein: Varies
Fat: Varies

Carbohydrates: Varies
Sugar: Varies

Pecans:
Calories: Approximately 7 calories per pecan half
Protein: 0.1g
Fat: 0.7g
Carbohydrates: 0.1g
Sugar: 0g

Low glycemic snacks

Baby Carrots with Hummus:
Calories: Approximately 10 calories per baby carrot
GI: Low (hummus may have a low to moderate GI)
GL: Low
Sugar: Varies by brand

Greek Yogurt (Plain, Non-fat) with Berries:
Calories: Approximately 100 per 6-ounce serving
GI: Low
GL: Low
Sugar: 4g (from natural sugars in yogurt and berries)

Cucumber Slices with Cream Cheese:
Calories: Varies, check product label
GI: Low
GL: Low
Sugar: Varies by brand

Nuts (e.g., Almonds, Walnuts):
Calories: Varies by type, refer to product label
GI: Low
GL: Low

Sugar: Varies by type

Cheese Cubes (e.g., Cheddar, Mozzarella):
Calories: Varies by type, refer to product label
GI: Low
GL: Low
Sugar: Varies by type

Hard-Boiled Eggs:
Calories: Approximately 68 per large egg
GI: Low
GL: Low
Sugar: 0g

Avocado Slices on Whole Grain Crackers:
Calories: Varies, check product label
GI: Low to moderate (crackers may affect GI)
GL: Varies
Sugar: Varies by brand

Cherry Tomatoes with Mozzarella Balls:
Calories: Varies, check product label
GI: Low
GL: Low
Sugar: Varies by brand

Apple Slices with Peanut Butter (No Added Sugar):
Calories: Varies, check product label
GI: Low
GL: Varies
Sugar: Varies by brand

Hummus with Whole Grain Pita Bread:
Calories: Varies, check product label
GI: Low to moderate
GL: Varies
Sugar: Varies by brand

Yogurt Parfait with Granola (No Added Sugar):
Calories: Varies, check product label
GI: Low (consider choosing low-GI granola)
GL: Varies
Sugar: Varies by brand

Celery Sticks with Almond Butter (No Added Sugar):
Calories: Varies, check product label
GI: Low
GL: Varies
Sugar: Varies by brand

Berries (e.g., Strawberries, Blueberries) with Cottage Cheese:
Calories: Varies, check product label
GI: Low
GL: Varies
Sugar: Varies by brand

Seaweed Snacks:
Calories: Approximately 20 per serving
GI: Low
GL: Low
Sugar: 0g

Sliced Bell Peppers with Guacamole:
Calories: Varies, check product label
GI: Low
GL: Varies
Sugar: Varies by brand

Low glycemic fats and oil

Olive Oil:
Calories: Approximately 120 per tablespoon
Total Fat: 14g
Saturated Fat: 2g
Unsaturated Fats: 10g (monounsaturated), 1.5g (polyunsaturated)
Trans Fat: 0g
Cholesterol: 0mg

Avocado:
Calories: Approximately 234 per avocado
Total Fat: 21g
Saturated Fat: 3g
Unsaturated Fats: 15g (monounsaturated), 2.7g (polyunsaturated)
Trans Fat: 0g
Cholesterol: 0mg

Coconut Oil:
Calories: Approximately 120 per tablespoon
Total Fat: 14g
Saturated Fat: 12g
Unsaturated Fats: 1.1g (monounsaturated), 0.2g (polyunsaturated)
Trans Fat: 0g
Cholesterol: 0mg

Almonds:
Calories: Approximately 7 calories per almond
Total Fat: 0.6g
Saturated Fat: 0.05g
Unsaturated Fats: 0.5g (monounsaturated), 0.1g (polyunsaturated)
Trans Fat: 0g
Cholesterol: 0mg

Walnuts:
Calories: Approximately 4 calories per walnut half
Total Fat: 0.4g
Saturated Fat: 0.04g
Unsaturated Fats: 0.3g (monounsaturated), 0.07g (polyunsaturated)
Trans Fat: 0g
Cholesterol: 0mg

Flaxseeds:
Calories: Approximately 37 calories per tablespoon (ground)
Total Fat: 3g
Saturated Fat: 0.3g
Unsaturated Fats: 2g (monounsaturated), 0.6g (polyunsaturated)
Trans Fat: 0g
Cholesterol: 0mg

Chia Seeds:
Calories: Approximately 69 calories per ounce
Total Fat: 4.4g
Saturated Fat: 0.4g

Unsaturated Fats: 3g (monounsaturated), 2g (polyunsaturated)
Trans Fat: 0g
Cholesterol: 0mg

Pumpkin Seeds (Pepitas):
Calories: Approximately 151 per ounce
Total Fat: 13g
Saturated Fat: 2.3g
Unsaturated Fats: 8.7g (monounsaturated), 1.9g (polyunsaturated)
Trans Fat: 0g
Cholesterol: 0mg

Cashews:
Calories: Approximately 8 calories per cashew
Total Fat: 0.6g
Saturated Fat: 0.12g
Unsaturated Fats: 0.4g (monounsaturated), 0.1g (polyunsaturated)
Trans Fat: 0g
Cholesterol: 0mg

Salmon (Wild-caught):
Calories: Approximately 206 per 3-ounce fillet
Total Fat: 13g
Saturated Fat: 2g
Unsaturated Fats: 7g (monounsaturated), 3g (polyunsaturated)
Trans Fat: 0g
Cholesterol: 68mg

Soybean Oil:
Calories: Approximately 120 per tablespoon
Total Fat: 14g
Saturated Fat: 2g
Unsaturated Fats: 8g (monounsaturated), 3.2g (polyunsaturated)
Trans Fat: 0g
Cholesterol: 0mg

Sunflower Oil:
Calories: Approximately 120 per tablespoon
Total Fat: 14g
Saturated Fat: 1.5g
Unsaturated Fats: 10g (monounsaturated), 3g (polyunsaturated)
Trans Fat: 0g
Cholesterol: 0mg

Peanut Butter (No Added Sugar):
Calories: Varies by brand, refer to product label
Total Fat: Varies
Saturated Fat: Varies
Unsaturated Fats: Varies
Trans Fat: 0g
Cholesterol: 0mg

Dark Chocolate (70-85% Cocoa):
Calories: Varies by brand, refer to product label
Total Fat: Varies
Saturated Fat: Varies
Unsaturated Fats: Varies
Trans Fat: 0g
Cholesterol: 0mg

Canola Oil:
Calories: Approximately 120 per tablespoon
Total Fat: 14g
Saturated Fat: 1g
Unsaturated Fats: 8g (monounsaturated), 4g (polyunsaturated)
Trans Fat: 0g
Cholesterol: 0mg

Low glycemic baking and cooking ingredients

Almond Flour:
Calories: Approximately 160 per 1/4 cup
GI: Low
GL: Low
Sugar: 0g

Coconut Flour:
Calories: Approximately 60 per 1/4 cup
GI: Low
GL: Low
Sugar: 3g

Stevia (Natural Sweetener):
Calories: Varies by brand, typically 0 per teaspoon
GI: Low
GL: Low
Sugar: 0g

Erythritol (Sugar Substitute):
Calories: Approximately 0.2 calories per gram (varies by brand)
GI: Low
GL: Low
Sugar: 0g

Flaxseed Meal:
Calories: Approximately 37 per tablespoon
GI: Low
GL: Low
Sugar: 0g

Chia Seeds:
Calories: Approximately 69 per ounce
GI: Low
GL: Low
Sugar: 0.2g

Whole Grain Oats:
Calories: Approximately 150 per 1/2 cup (dry)
GI: Low to moderate (varies with processing)
GL: Varies
Sugar: 1g

Quinoa:
Calories: Approximately 111 per 1/2 cup (cooked)
GI: Low
GL: Low
Sugar: 1.5g

Cocoa Powder (Unsweetened):
Calories: Approximately 12 per tablespoon

GI: Low
GL: Low
Sugar: 0.1g

Unsweetened Applesauce:
Calories: Approximately 50 per 1/2 cup
GI: Low
GL: Low
Sugar: 9g (natural sugars)

Coconut Oil:
Calories: Approximately 120 per tablespoon
GI: Does not apply (no carbohydrates)
GL: Does not apply
Sugar: 0g

Baking Powder (Aluminum-Free):
Calories: Varies by brand, typically 0
GI: Does not apply
GL: Does not apply
Sugar: 0g

Vinegar (e.g., Apple Cider Vinegar):
Calories: Varies, typically 0
GI: Low
GL: Low
Sugar: 0g

Cinnamon:
Calories: Varies, typically 0
GI: Low
GL: Low
Sugar: 0g

Unsweetened Nut Butters (e.g., Almond Butter, Peanut Butter):
Calories: Varies by brand, refer to product label
GI: Low
GL: Low
Sugar: Varies

Low glycemic beverages

Water:
Calories: 0
GI: Does not apply (no carbohydrates)
GL: Does not apply
Sugar: 0g

Herbal Tea (Unsweetened):
Calories: 0
GI: Does not apply (no carbohydrates)
GL: Does not apply
Sugar: 0g

Green Tea (Unsweetened):
Calories: 0
GI: Does not apply (no carbohydrates)
GL: Does not apply
Sugar: 0g

Black Coffee (Unsweetened):
Calories: 2 per 8-ounce cup
GI: Does not apply (no carbohydrates)
GL: Does not apply
Sugar: 0g

Sparkling Water (Unsweetened):
Calories: 0
GI: Does not apply (no carbohydrates)
GL: Does not apply
Sugar: 0g

Vegetable Juice (Low-Sodium, Unsweetened):
Calories: Varies, check product label
GI: Low
GL: Varies
Sugar: Varies by brand

Almond Milk (Unsweetened):
Calories: Approximately 30 per cup
GI: Low
GL: Low
Sugar: 0g

Coconut Water (Unsweetened):
Calories: Approximately 46 per cup
GI: Low to moderate
GL: Varies
Sugar: 6g

Lemonade (Homemade with Stevia):
Calories: Varies, check recipe
GI: Low
GL: Varies
Sugar: 0g

Tomato Juice (Low-Sodium, Unsweetened):
Calories: Varies, check product label
GI: Low

GL: Varies
Sugar: Varies by brand

Iced Herbal Tea (Unsweetened):
Calories: 0
GI: Does not apply (no carbohydrates)
GL: Does not apply
Sugar: 0g

Unsweetened Soy Milk:
Calories: Varies, check product label
GI: Low
GL: Varies
Sugar: Varies by brand

Kombucha (Unsweetened):
Calories: Varies, check product label
GI: Low
GL: Varies
Sugar: Varies by brand

Whey Protein Shake (Unsweetened):
Calories: Varies, check product label
GI: Low
GL: Varies
Sugar: Varies by brand

Unsweetened Greek Yogurt Smoothie:
Calories: Varies, check product label
GI: Low
GL: Varies
Sugar: Varies by brand

Low glycemic condiments and sauces

Mustard:
Calories: Approximately 3 per tablespoon
GI: Low
GL: Low
Sugar: 0g

Vinegar (e.g., Balsamic, Apple Cider):
Calories: Varies, typically 0
GI: Low
GL: Low
Sugar: 0g

Soy Sauce (Reduced Sodium):
Calories: Approximately 10 per tablespoon
GI: Low
GL: Low
Sugar: 1g

Hot Sauce (e.g., Tabasco):
Calories: Varies, typically 0
GI: Low
GL: Low
Sugar: 0g

Pesto Sauce (Homemade or Low-Sugar Store-Bought):
Calories: Varies, check product label
GI: Low
GL: Varies
Sugar: Varies

Guacamole:
Calories: Varies, check product label or make homemade
GI: Low
GL: Varies
Sugar: Varies

Tahini:
Calories: Approximately 89 per tablespoon
GI: Low
GL: Low
Sugar: 0g

Salsa (Homemade or Low-Sugar Store-Bought):
Calories: Varies, check product label or make homemade
GI: Low
GL: Varies
Sugar: Varies

Hummus (Low-Sugar Varieties):
Calories: Varies, check product label
GI: Low to moderate
GL: Varies
Sugar: Varies

Worcestershire Sauce (Reduced Sodium):
Calories: Approximately 5 per teaspoon
GI: Low
GL: Low
Sugar: 1g

Peanut Sauce (Homemade or Low-Sugar Store-Bought):
Calories: Varies, check product label or make homemade
GI: Low
GL: Varies
Sugar: Varies

Low-Fat Greek Yogurt Dressing:
Calories: Varies, check product label
GI: Low
GL: Varies
Sugar: Varies

Olive Tapenade:
Calories: Varies, check product label or make homemade
GI: Low
GL: Varies
Sugar: Varies

Low-Sugar Barbecue Sauce:
Calories: Varies, check product label or make homemade
GI: Low to moderate
GL: Varies
Sugar: Varies

Low-Fat Salad Dressing (Vinaigrette, Italian, etc.):
Calories: Varies, check product label
GI: Low
GL: Varies
Sugar: Varies

Low glycemic Dressing and marinades

Olive Oil and Balsamic Vinegar Dressing:
Calories: Approximately 120 per tablespoon
GI: Low
GL: Low
Sugar: 0g

Greek Yogurt and Lemon Dressing:
Calories: Varies, check product label or make homemade
GI: Low
GL: Varies
Sugar: Varies

Tahini and Lemon Marinade:
Calories: Approximately 89 per tablespoon
GI: Low
GL: Low
Sugar: 0g

Mustard and Herb Vinaigrette:
Calories: Varies, check product label or make homemade
GI: Low
GL: Varies
Sugar: Varies

Avocado and Lime Dressing:
Calories: Varies, check product label or make homemade
GI: Low
GL: Varies
Sugar: Varies

Soy Ginger Marinade (Reduced Sodium):
Calories: Varies, check product label or make homemade
GI: Low
GL: Varies
Sugar: Varies

Cilantro Lime Yogurt Dressing:
Calories: Varies, check product label or make homemade
GI: Low
GL: Varies
Sugar: Varies

Balsamic Glaze (Reduced Sugar):
Calories: Varies, check product label or make homemade
GI: Low
GL: Varies
Sugar: Varies

Lemon Garlic Herb Marinade:
Calories: Varies, check product label or make homemade
GI: Low
GL: Varies
Sugar: Varies

Cider Vinegar and Dijon Mustard Dressing:
Calories: Varies, check product label or make homemade
GI: Low
GL: Varies

Sugar: Varies

Yogurt Ranch Dressing (Low-Fat):
Calories: Varies, check product label or make homemade
GI: Low
GL: Varies
Sugar: Varies

Pesto Sauce (Homemade or Low-Sugar Store-Bought):
Calories: Varies, check product label or make homemade
GI: Low
GL: Varies
Sugar: Varies

Lemon Dill Yogurt Sauce:
Calories: Varies, check product label or make homemade
GI: Low
GL: Varies
Sugar: Varies

Tomato Basil Vinaigrette:
Calories: Varies, check product label or make homemade
GI: Low
GL: Varies
Sugar: Varies

Sesame Ginger Dressing (Reduced Sodium):
Calories: Varies, check product label or make
homemade
GI: Low
GL: Varies
Sugar: Varies

Low glycemic herbs and spices

Cinnamon:
Calories: Varies (negligible)
GI: Low
GL: Low
Sugar: 0g

Turmeric:
Calories: Varies (negligible)
GI: Low
GL: Low
Sugar: 0g

Cayenne Pepper:
Calories: Varies (negligible)
GI: Low
GL: Low
Sugar: 0g

Ginger:
Calories: Varies (negligible)
GI: Low
GL: Low
Sugar: 0g

Basil:
Calories: Varies (negligible)
GI: Low
GL: Low
Sugar: 0g

Oregano:
Calories: Varies (negligible)
GI: Low
GL: Low
Sugar: 0g

Rosemary:
Calories: Varies (negligible)
GI: Low
GL: Low
Sugar: 0g

Thyme:
Calories: Varies (negligible)
GI: Low
GL: Low
Sugar: 0g

Coriander (Cilantro):
Calories: Varies (negligible)
GI: Low
GL: Low
Sugar: 0g

Garlic Powder:
Calories: Varies (negligible)
GI: Low

GL: Low
Sugar: 0g

Cumin:
Calories: Varies (negligible)
GI: Low
GL: Low
Sugar: 0g

Paprika:
Calories: Varies (negligible)
GI: Low
GL: Low
Sugar: 0g

Sage:
Calories: Varies (negligible)
GI: Low
GL: Low
Sugar: 0g

Mint:
Calories: Varies (negligible)
GI: Low
GL: Low
Sugar: 0g

Cilantro (Fresh Coriander):
Calories: Varies (negligible)
GI: Low
GL: Low
Sugar: 0g

Guacamole:
Calories: Varies, check product label or make homemade
GI: Low
GL: Varies
Sugar: Varies

Hummus (Low-Sugar Varieties):
Calories: Varies, check product label
GI: Low to moderate
GL: Varies
Sugar: Varies

Salsa (Homemade or Low-Sugar Store-Bought):
Calories: Varies, check product label or make homemade
GI: Low
GL: Varies
Sugar: Varies

Peanut Butter (No Added Sugar):
Calories: Varies by brand, refer to product label
GI: Low
GL: Varies
Sugar: Varies

Greek Yogurt Dip (Low-Fat):
Calories: Varies, check product label
GI: Low
GL: Varies
Sugar: Varies

Sour Cream (Reduced Fat):
Calories: Varies, check product label
GI: Low
GL: Varies
Sugar: Varies

Cream Cheese (Low-Fat):
Calories: Varies, check product label
GI: Low
GL: Varies
Sugar: Varies

Almond Butter (No Added Sugar):
Calories: Varies by brand, refer to product label
GI: Low
GL: Varies
Sugar: Varies

Tzatziki Sauce:
Calories: Varies, check product label or make homemade
GI: Low
GL: Varies
Sugar: Varies

Olive Tapenade:
Calories: Varies, check product label or make homemade
GI: Low
GL: Varies
Sugar: Varies

Pesto Sauce (Homemade or Low-Sugar Store-Bought):
Calories: Varies, check product label or make homemade
GI: Low
GL: Varies
Sugar: Varies

Cottage Cheese (Low-Fat):
Calories: Varies, check product label
GI: Low
GL: Varies
Sugar: Varies

Tahini:
Calories: Approximately 89 per tablespoon
GI: Low
GL: Low
Sugar: 0g

Lemon Garlic Hummus:
Calories: Varies, check product label or make homemade
GI: Low to moderate
GL: Varies
Sugar: Varies

Avocado Salsa:
Calories: Varies, check product label or make homemade
GI: Low
GL: Varies
Sugar: Varies

Low glycemic sweeteners

Stevia:
Calories: 0
GI: Low
GL: Low
Sugar: 0g

Erythritol:
Calories: 0.2 calories per gram (varies by brand)
GI: Low
GL: Low
Sugar: 0g

Monk Fruit Extract:
Calories: 0
GI: Low
GL: Low
Sugar: 0g

Xylitol:
Calories: Approximately 2.4 calories per gram
GI: Low
GL: Low
Sugar: 0g

Agave Nectar (in moderation):
Calories: Approximately 21 per teaspoon
GI: Low
GL: Low to moderate
Sugar: 5g

Allulose:
Calories: Approximately 0.4 calories per gram
GI: Low
GL: Low
Sugar: 0g

Inulin-based Sweeteners (Chicory Root):
Calories: Varies, check product label
GI: Low
GL: Varies
Sugar: Varies

Yacon Syrup:
Calories: Varies, check product label
GI: Low
GL: Varies
Sugar: Varies

Coconut Sugar:
Calories: Approximately 15 per teaspoon
GI: Low to moderate
GL: Low to moderate
Sugar: 4g

Tagatose:
Calories: Approximately 1.5 calories per gram
GI: Low
GL: Low
Sugar: 0g

Lucuma Powder:
Calories: Varies, check product label
GI: Low

GL: Varies
Sugar: Varies

Stevia Blends (Erythritol-Stevia, Monk Fruit-Stevia):
Calories: Varies, check product label
GI: Low
GL: Varies
Sugar: Varies

Date Sugar (Use sparingly):
Calories: Approximately 11 per teaspoon
GI: Low to moderate
GL: Low to moderate
Sugar: 2.8g

Maltitol:
Calories: Approximately 2.1 calories per gram
GI: Low to moderate
GL: Low to moderate
Sugar: 0g

Sucralose (Splenda):
Calories: 3.36 calories per gram
GI: Low
GL: Low
Sugar: 0g

Breakfast Recipes

1. Quinoa and Berry Breakfast Bowl:
Ingredients:
1/2 cup quinoa (rinsed)
1 cup mixed berries (strawberries, blueberries, raspberries)
1 tablespoon chia seeds
1 tablespoon almond butter
1 teaspoon honey (optional)

Preparation:
Cook quinoa according to package instructions.
In a bowl, mix cooked quinoa, berries, chia seeds, and almond butter.
Drizzle with honey if desired.
Nutritional Information (Per Serving):
Calories: ~300
GI Value: Low
GI Load: Low
Sugar: Varies based on fruit and honey usage

2. Greek Yogurt Parfait:
Ingredients:
1 cup Greek yogurt (unsweetened)
1/2 cup granola (choose low-sugar options)
1/2 cup mixed berries
1 tablespoon chopped nuts (almonds, walnuts)

Preparation:
In a glass, layer Greek yogurt, granola, berries, and nuts.
Repeat the layers.
Top with a few extra berries and nuts.
Nutritional Information (Per Serving):
Calories: ~350
GI Value: Low
GI Load: Low
Sugar: Varies based on yogurt and granola choice

3. Sweet Potato and Spinach Breakfast Wrap:
Ingredients:
1 medium sweet potato (grated)
2 eggs (whisked)
1 cup fresh spinach
Whole-grain tortilla
Salt and pepper to taste

Preparation:
Sauté grated sweet potato in a pan until softened.
Add fresh spinach and cook until wilted.
Pour whisked eggs over the vegetables and scramble until cooked.
Place the mixture on a whole-grain tortilla, season with salt and pepper, and wrap.
Nutritional Information (Per Serving):
Calories: ~300
GI Value: Low
GI Load: Low
Sugar: Minimal

4. Chia Seed Pudding:
Ingredients:
2 tablespoons chia seeds
1 cup unsweetened almond milk
1/2 teaspoon vanilla extract
Fresh fruit for topping (e.g., berries, kiwi)

Preparation:
Mix chia seeds, almond milk, and vanilla extract in a
bowl.
Refrigerate for at least 2 hours or overnight until a
pudding consistency is reached.
Top with fresh fruit before serving.
Nutritional Information (Per Serving):
Calories: ~150
GI Value: Low
GI Load: Low
Sugar: Varies based on fruit topping

5. Egg and Veggie Muffin Cups:
Ingredients:
4 eggs
1/2 cup diced bell peppers
1/2 cup diced tomatoes
1/4 cup diced onions
Salt and pepper to taste

Preparation:
Preheat the oven to 350°F (175°C).
In a bowl, whisk eggs and season with salt and
pepper.
Grease a muffin tin and distribute diced vegetables
evenly.

Pour whisked eggs over the vegetables.
Bake for 15-20 minutes until eggs are set.
Nutritional Information (Per Serving):
Calories: ~120
GI Value: Low
GI Load: Low
Sugar: Minimal

Lunch Recipes

1. Grilled Salmon with Quinoa and Roasted Vegetables:
Ingredients:
6 oz salmon fillet
1/2 cup quinoa (rinsed)
Mixed vegetables (e.g., bell peppers, zucchini, cherry tomatoes)
Olive oil, lemon juice, salt, and pepper for seasoning

Preparation:
Marinate salmon with olive oil, lemon juice, salt, and pepper.
Grill salmon until cooked through.
Roast mixed vegetables in the oven.
Cook quinoa according to package instructions.
Serve grilled salmon on a bed of quinoa with roasted vegetables on the side.
Nutritional Information (Per Serving):
Calories: ~400
GI Value: Low
GI Load: Low
Sugar: Minimal

2. Chickpea and Vegetable Stir-Fry:
Ingredients:
1 cup cooked chickpeas
Mixed vegetables (e.g., broccoli, bell peppers, snap peas)
2 tablespoons low-sodium soy sauce
1 tablespoon sesame oil
Brown rice (cooked)

Preparation:
Sauté mixed vegetables in sesame oil until slightly tender.
Add cooked chickpeas and soy sauce to the pan.
Stir-fry until everything is well-coated and heated through.
Serve over a bed of brown rice.
Nutritional Information (Per Serving):
Calories: ~350
GI Value: Low
GI Load: Low
Sugar: Minimal

3. Mushroom and Spinach Quiche with Whole Wheat Crust:
Ingredients:
Whole wheat pie crust
1 cup sliced mushrooms
2 cups fresh spinach
4 eggs
1 cup low-fat milk
Salt, pepper, and herbs for seasoning

Preparation:
Preheat the oven to 375°F (190°C).
Sauté mushrooms and spinach until wilted.
In a bowl, whisk together eggs, milk, salt, pepper, and herbs.
Pour the egg mixture into the pie crust and add sautéed vegetables.
Bake for 30-35 minutes until set.
Nutritional Information (Per Serving):
Calories: ~300
GI Value: Low
GI Load: Low
Sugar: Minimal

4. Turkey and Vegetable Lettuce Wraps:
Ingredients:
Ground turkey
Lettuce leaves (e.g., iceberg or butter lettuce)
Mixed vegetables (e.g., carrots, bell peppers, water chestnuts)
Low-sodium soy sauce, ginger, and garlic for seasoning

Preparation:
Cook ground turkey in a pan until browned.
Add mixed vegetables, soy sauce, ginger, and garlic to the pan.
Stir until vegetables are tender.
Spoon the mixture onto lettuce leaves and wrap.
Nutritional Information (Per Serving):
Calories: ~250
GI Value: Low
GI Load: Low

Sugar: Minimal

5. Quinoa Salad with Chickpeas and Feta:
Ingredients:
1 cup cooked quinoa (rinsed)
1 cup canned chickpeas (drained and rinsed)
Cherry tomatoes, cucumber, red onion (diced)
Feta cheese (crumbled)
Olive oil, lemon juice, salt, and pepper for dressing

Preparation:
In a large bowl, combine quinoa, chickpeas, tomatoes, cucumber, and red onion.
Drizzle with olive oil and lemon juice, season with salt and pepper.
Toss until well mixed.
Sprinkle feta cheese on top before serving.
Nutritional Information (Per Serving):
Calories: ~350
GI Value: Low
GI Load: Low
Sugar: Minimal

1. Grilled Chicken with Quinoa and Roasted Vegetables:
Ingredients:
6 oz chicken breast
1/2 cup quinoa (rinsed)
Mixed vegetables (e.g., asparagus, bell peppers, cherry tomatoes)
Olive oil, lemon juice, garlic, salt, and pepper for seasoning

Preparation:
Marinate chicken with olive oil, lemon juice, garlic, salt, and pepper.
Grill chicken until cooked through.
Roast mixed vegetables in the oven.
Cook quinoa according to package instructions.
Serve grilled chicken on a bed of quinoa with roasted vegetables on the side.
Nutritional Information (Per Serving):
Calories: ~400
GI Value: Low
GI Load: Low
Sugar: Minimal

2. Salmon and Asparagus Foil Packets:
Ingredients:
6 oz salmon fillet
Asparagus spears
Lemon slices
Olive oil, garlic, dill, salt, and pepper for seasoning

Preparation:
Preheat the oven to 375°F (190°C).
Place salmon fillet on a sheet of foil.
Arrange asparagus around the salmon, add lemon slices, and season with olive oil, garlic, dill, salt, and pepper.
Seal the foil into packets and bake for 20-25 minutes.
Nutritional Information (Per Serving):
Calories: ~350
GI Value: Low
GI Load: Low
Sugar: Minimal

3. Vegetarian Lentil Soup:
Ingredients:
1 cup dried green or brown lentils (rinsed)
Carrots, celery, onion, and garlic (chopped)
Vegetable broth
Cumin, coriander, turmeric, salt, and pepper for seasoning

Preparation:
Sauté chopped vegetables in a pot until softened.
Add lentils, vegetable broth, and seasonings.
Simmer for 30-40 minutes until lentils are tender.
Adjust seasoning as needed before serving.
Nutritional Information (Per Serving):
Calories: ~300
GI Value: Low
GI Load: Low
Sugar: Minimal

4. Eggplant and Chickpea Curry:
Ingredients:
1 medium eggplant (cubed)
1 can chickpeas (drained and rinsed)
Coconut milk
Curry powder, cumin, coriander, turmeric, garlic,
and ginger for seasoning

Preparation:
Sauté cubed eggplant until lightly browned.
Add chickpeas, coconut milk, and seasonings.
Simmer until the eggplant is tender and the flavors
meld.
Serve over brown rice or quinoa.
Nutritional Information (Per Serving):
Calories: ~350
GI Value: Low
GI Load: Low
Sugar: Minimal

5. Turkey and Vegetable Stir-Fry with Brown Rice:
Ingredients:
Ground turkey
Mixed vegetables (e.g., broccoli, bell peppers, snap
peas)
Low-sodium soy sauce, ginger, and garlic for
seasoning
Brown rice (cooked)

Preparation:
Cook ground turkey in a pan until browned.
Add mixed vegetables, soy sauce, ginger, and garlic
to the pan.

Stir-fry until everything is well-coated and heated through.
Serve over a bed of brown rice.
Nutritional Information (Per Serving):
Calories: ~300
GI Value: Low
GI Load: Low
Sugar: Minimal

Desserts Recipes

1. Chia Seed Pudding with Berries:
Ingredients:
2 tablespoons chia seeds
1 cup unsweetened almond milk
1/2 teaspoon vanilla extract
Mixed berries (e.g., strawberries, blueberries)

Preparation:
Mix chia seeds, almond milk, and vanilla extract in a bowl.
Refrigerate for at least 2 hours or overnight until a pudding consistency is reached.
Top with mixed berries before serving.
Nutritional Information (Per Serving):
Calories: ~150
GI Value: Low
GI Load: Low
Sugar: Varies based on fruit topping

2. Baked Apples with Cinnamon and Walnuts:
Ingredients:
Apples (sliced)
Cinnamon

Chopped walnuts
1 tablespoon honey (optional)

Preparation:
Preheat the oven to 375°F (190°C).
Arrange apple slices in a baking dish.
Sprinkle with cinnamon and chopped walnuts.
Drizzle with honey if desired.
Bake for 20-25 minutes until apples are tender.
Nutritional Information (Per Serving):
Calories: ~120
GI Value: Low
GI Load: Low
Sugar: Varies based on honey usage

3. Greek Yogurt Parfait with Nuts and Berries:
Ingredients:
1 cup Greek yogurt (unsweetened)
Mixed berries (e.g., raspberries, blackberries)
Chopped nuts (e.g., almonds, walnuts)
1 teaspoon honey (optional)

Preparation:
In a glass, layer Greek yogurt, mixed berries, and chopped nuts.
Repeat the layers.
Drizzle with honey if desired.
Nutritional Information (Per Serving):
Calories: ~250
GI Value: Low
GI Load: Low
Sugar: Varies based on honey usage

4. Dark Chocolate Avocado Mousse:
Ingredients:
2 ripe avocados
1/4 cup unsweetened cocoa powder
1/4 cup maple syrup or agave nectar
1 teaspoon vanilla extract

Preparation:
Blend avocados, cocoa powder, maple syrup, and vanilla extract in a food processor until smooth.
Refrigerate for at least 30 minutes before serving.
Nutritional Information (Per Serving):
Calories: ~200
GI Value: Low
GI Load: Low
Sugar: Varies based on sweetener choice

5. Berries and Cream Parfait:
Ingredients:
Mixed berries (e.g., strawberries, blueberries, raspberries)
Low-fat whipped cream or Greek yogurt
1 tablespoon chopped nuts (e.g., pistachios, almonds)

Preparation:
In a glass, layer mixed berries and a dollop of low-fat whipped cream or Greek yogurt.
Repeat the layers.
Top with chopped nuts before serving.
Nutritional Information (Per Serving):
Calories: ~180
GI Value: Low

GI Load: Low
Sugar: Varies based on yogurt or whipped cream choice

Smoothies Recipes

1. Berry Bliss Smoothie:
Ingredients:
1/2 cup mixed berries (strawberries, blueberries, raspberries)
1/2 banana (frozen for creaminess)
1/2 cup Greek yogurt (unsweetened)
1 tablespoon chia seeds
1/2 cup unsweetened almond milk

Preparation:
Blend all ingredients until smooth.
Adjust consistency with more almond milk if needed.
Nutritional Information (Per Serving):
Calories: ~200
GI Value: Low
GI Load: Low
Sugar: Varies based on fruit ripeness

2. Green Power Smoothie:
Ingredients:
1 cup spinach or kale
1/2 cucumber
1/2 green apple
1/2 avocado
1 tablespoon flaxseeds
1/2 cup coconut water

Preparation:
Blend all ingredients until smooth.
Add more coconut water if a thinner consistency is desired.
Nutritional Information (Per Serving):
Calories: ~250
GI Value: Low
GI Load: Low
Sugar: Varies based on fruit ripeness

3. Cocoa Almond Delight:
Ingredients:
1 tablespoon unsweetened cocoa powder
1/2 banana (frozen for creaminess)
1 tablespoon almond butter
1/2 cup low-fat Greek yogurt
1/2 cup unsweetened almond milk

Preparation:
Blend all ingredients until smooth.
Adjust thickness with more almond milk if necessary.
Nutritional Information (Per Serving):
Calories: ~250
GI Value: Low
GI Load: Low
Sugar: Varies based on fruit ripeness

4. Peachy Keen Protein Smoothie:
Ingredients:
1/2 cup frozen peaches
1/2 cup cottage cheese (low-fat)
1 scoop vanilla protein powder

1 tablespoon honey (optional)
1/2 cup water or unsweetened almond milk

Preparation:
Blend all ingredients until smooth.
Add more liquid for desired consistency.
Nutritional Information (Per Serving):
Calories: ~300
GI Value: Low
GI Load: Low
Sugar: Varies based on fruit ripeness and honey usage

5. Tropical Paradise Smoothie:
Ingredients:
1/2 cup pineapple chunks
1/2 banana (frozen for creaminess)
1/2 cup coconut water
1/2 cup low-fat Greek yogurt
1 tablespoon chia seeds

Preparation:
Blend all ingredients until smooth.
Adjust thickness with more coconut water if needed.
Nutritional Information (Per Serving):
Calories: ~220
GI Value: Low
GI Load: Low
Sugar: Varies based on fruit ripeness

1. Roasted Chickpeas:
Ingredients:
1 can chickpeas (drained and rinsed)
1 tablespoon olive oil
1 teaspoon smoked paprika
1/2 teaspoon garlic powder
Salt to taste

Preparation:
Preheat the oven to 400°F (200°C).
Toss chickpeas with olive oil, smoked paprika, garlic powder, and salt.
Roast for 25-30 minutes until crispy.
Nutritional Information (Per Serving):
Calories: ~150
GI Value: Low
GI Load: Low
Sugar: Minimal

2. Greek Yogurt with Berries and Nuts:
Ingredients:
1/2 cup Greek yogurt (unsweetened)
Mixed berries (e.g., strawberries, blueberries)
1 tablespoon chopped nuts (e.g., almonds, walnuts)
1 teaspoon honey (optional)

Preparation:
In a bowl, layer Greek yogurt, mixed berries, and chopped nuts.
Drizzle with honey if desired.
Nutritional Information (Per Serving):
Calories: ~200

GI Value: Low
GI Load: Low
Sugar: Varies based on fruit ripeness and honey usage

3. Vegetable Sticks with Hummus:
Ingredients:
Carrot, cucumber, and bell pepper sticks
1/4 cup hummus (low-fat)

Preparation:
Cut vegetables into sticks.
Serve with a side of hummus for dipping.
Nutritional Information (Per Serving):
Calories: ~100
GI Value: Low
GI Load: Low
Sugar: Minimal

4. Cheese and Whole Grain Crackers:
Ingredients:
Whole grain crackers
Cheese slices (e.g., cheddar, mozzarella)

Preparation:
Arrange whole grain crackers with cheese slices.
Nutritional Information (Per Serving):
Calories: ~150
GI Value: Low
GI Load: Low
Sugar: Minimal

5. Trail Mix with Nuts and Seeds:
Ingredients:
Almonds, walnuts, sunflower seeds, pumpkin seeds
Dried berries (e.g., cranberries, blueberries)
Dark chocolate chips (optional)

Preparation:
Mix nuts, seeds, and dried berries in a bowl.
Add dark chocolate chips if desired.
Nutritional Information (Per Serving):
Calories: ~200
GI Value: Low
GI Load: Low
Sugar: Varies based on dried fruit and chocolate usage

CONCLUSION

In conclusion, crafting a well-thought-out grocery and food list for individuals with Type 2 Diabetes is a crucial step towards managing the condition effectively. The emphasis on nutrient-dense, low-glycemic, and balanced food choices can play a pivotal role in stabilizing blood sugar levels, promoting overall health, and preventing complications associated with diabetes. From non-starchy vegetables to lean protein sources, healthy fats, whole grains, and carefully selected fruits, each item on the list serves a purpose in supporting optimal nutritional needs.

Moreover, understanding the glycemic index, load, and other nutritional details empowers individuals to make informed decisions about their dietary intake. The focus on portion control, mindful eating, and maintaining a healthy weight further contributes to successful diabetes management.

It's essential for individuals with Type 2 Diabetes to collaborate with healthcare professionals, including dietitians, to tailor their grocery and food choices to their specific health needs and preferences. Regular monitoring of blood sugar levels, coupled with a commitment to a well-rounded, diabetes-friendly diet, forms the foundation for achieving better overall well-being and preventing long-term complications.

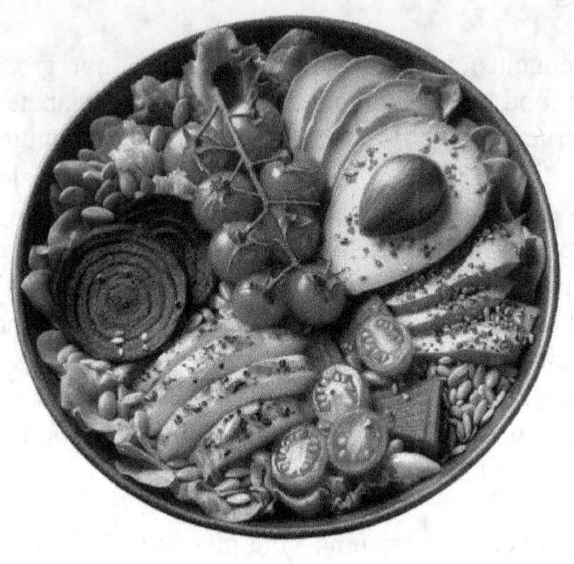

I trust this culinary journey has not only ignited your passion for wholesome eating but has also become a haven of inspiration, solace, and invaluable insights. Each carefully curated recipe within this type 2 diabetic grocery and food list reflects a dedication to excellence, with a profound understanding of the comprehensive guide to the type 2 diabetic grocery and food list.

Crafted with meticulous attention to detail, these recipes go beyond the realm of mere sustenance; they are a testament to the art of nourishing the body and soul. Your reviews, experiences, and insights are treasures that guide me on this culinary odyssey.

Every evaluation is a stepping stone for refinement, as I aspire to tailor this food list to surpass your expectations. Let's engage in a dialogue that transcends the pages, creating a connection that resonates with your culinary preferences and well-being goals.

Warm Culinary Regards,

Tina Feldman